The Best Natural Healing Tips

The Best Natural Healing Tips

Dr Sean Murphy

ISBN: 1544140134
ISBN 13: 9781544140131

For my Dad, Garry Robert Murphy

INTRODUCTION

"While other professions are concerned with changing the environment to suit the weakened body, chiropractic is concerned with strengthening the body to suit the environment."
— B. J. PALMER

As I sit down to write out the top healing tips, I must tell you that by no means is this list extensive, but it is REAL. My attempt on the television show as well as within this book is to give you something to think about that perhaps you have not thought of in the past. My goal is to go deeper and give amazing insider information that can only be gained by working in a clinical setting for 20 years as I have. These tips will hopefully inspire you and at times may even make you smile. Joy and laughter are important in life, and where possible I have interjected some of my own humour, because life is funny after all.

These natural tips have been tested clinically and have been proven to help in most cases. While many tips have not necessarily been tested in a research laboratory setting, it is my belief that the best laboratory is real life with real people. Scientific research is always behind the times and usually only proves something we already knew for many years. In modern times, we are identifying that many 'scientific proofs' are flawed and often influenced by a financial gain or bias (but that's a story for another book).

My education has been, not only in the most powerful human function, but also the resolutions to the nagging, everyday problems we all face. I have cared for the needs of highly influential people in the world, but my heart's desire is to help people living life in *real* time with *real* issues. Pains, stressors, discomfort, fear, anxiety, stress, depression, and relationship breakdown are all part of THIS real life.

Thank you for starting fresh. Thank you for taking a step towards a better, healthier, more powerful YOU. For more information on any of the tips in this book, please go to our Blog page (www.murphyhealthcentre.com/blog). On the site, we have listed ALL the video clips from our CTV Morning Live segments as well as more recently, our CTV Noon News appearances. I hope you find the answers to some of your questions here, and if not, tune in to the television show this year and get your questions answered LIVE.

Bless you,
Dr. Sean

CHAPTER 1

GAINING DAILY COMFORT

"You have to leave the city of your comfort and go into the wilderness of your intuition. What you'll discover will be wonderful. What you'll discover is yourself."
– ALAN ALDA

E very day we submit ourselves to stressful environments that force our bodies out of correct posture. Sitting, standing or laying still for long periods of time can cause postural deformities that lead to spinal irritation and a loss of good health. To regain your daily comfort, we need to look at some of the scenarios that require you to be in a specific position for a lengthy period of time and what you can do to help.

Driving Comfort

A long drive will force you to sit still and concentrate on the task at hand; which is driving safely to your destination. Most people don't stop and pull over for many (or any) breaks along the way, so I have included an easy tip here to help you keep on truckin' in comfort.

Bring a beach towel for behind your back and keep your head against the head rest. Fold the beach towel in many different ways and as you drive your passenger can change the towel fold and replace it behind your back. The secret to comfort as you drive is to change your position many times and remember to take fresh air breaks along the way. Your fresh air break may be simply rolling down the window for a few minutes, but the best fresh air break is to pull over, get out and walk around for ten minutes. Do this once every hour.

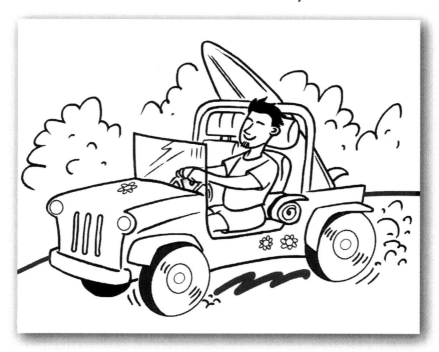

Desk Comfort

Use a stand-up desk. You can find inexpensive yet quality stand-up desks at any Canadian or Swedish furniture store and slightly more expensive versions at any Canadian office supply store.

If a stand-up desk is not an option, raise your computer up to eye level. Be sure to have a desk chair that can move up and down throughout the day. If studying from a book, use a holder for your book that tips it up and place it on top of one or two other text books bringing your reader to eye level.

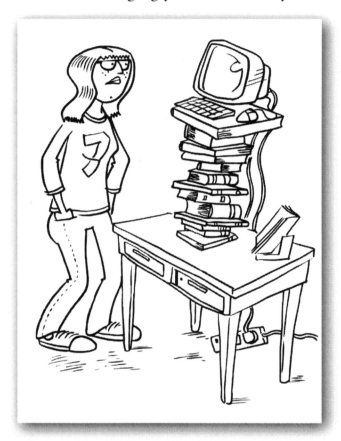

Doctor's tip... Like driving comfort already mentioned, re-member to change your position many times throughout the day and take fresh air breaks (avoid the smoking section at work). Regular, refreshing movement is very important for your posture. Your body is designed to move. Getting into the bad habit of sitting still at your desk or in your car is *very* destructive to your spine and brain. Remember, 90% of the nutrition for your brain comes from movement of the spine, so be sure to move frequently.

Sleep Comfort

Sleep on your belly-side or back-side by using a standard pillow and a body pillow. Place the body pillow along your side lengthways and use your other pillow normally. The body pillow will enable you to 'lean' forward or lay backwards on it, while the other pillow supports your head. When you lean forward or backwards with the body pillow, you avoid the torque that is normally created from twisting your neck to breath. If you are regularly a side sleeper, adding the body pillow will allow you to tilt off of the sharps points of your shoulder and hips.

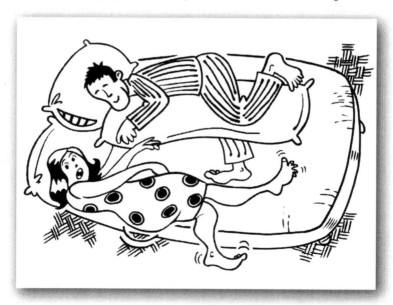

Doctor's tip... This body pillow sleeping tip comes from the many nights I realized that the couch can be more comfortable than my bed. On the nights I slept on the couch, I would wake up feeling refreshed, rested, with no pain or stiffness. I wondered why this was happening then it hit me...I CAN LEAN!! The shape of the couch allowed me to lean back against the backrest of the couch while my head remained supported on my pillow.

In order to create this scenario in my bed (to also salvage the relationship with my amazing wife) I decided to use a body pillow to create the lean-to and voila, the same couch-type setting was created and a resultant restful sleep.

Pillow Comfort

The best pillow you can own is one you can fluff up or compress. Your pillow should be able to 'change' to be effective. It should have stuffing that allows you to fluff the pillow up or squish it flat. Your pillow should also be designed for your size and stature as well. Bigger people may require a bigger, fuller pillow, whereas smaller people might need a flatter pillow.

Your pillow and mattress have to blend as well. You may need a soft pillow combined with a firm mattress depending on your size. Some other people may need a firm pillow with a soft mattress. You decide what works best - try different combinations until you get it right.

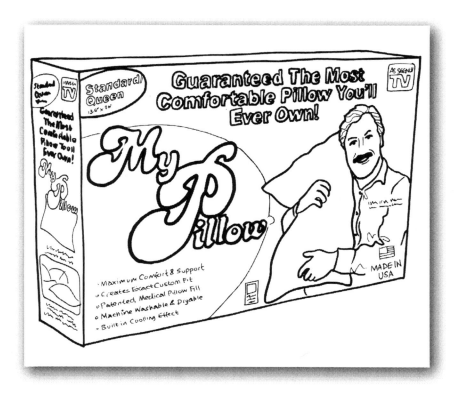

Doctor's tip... My favourite pillow (and I don't get paid for saying this) is called, "My Pillow". This pillow has pieces of foam all cut up inside it and you can change the thickness simply by fluffing it up or squishing it down.

Despite the silly picture of the man on the box, "My Pillow" is a very good pillow produced by Mike Lindell (the guy with the moustache on the box). The company is so sure you will love the pillow, it is guaranteed to be *"The most comfortable pillow you will ever own"* (that means you can return it if you don't like it and I like that policy!)

Sitting Comfort

Your chair and couch at home should allow you to rest your head comfortably against the back of the couch, like the headrests in your car. Your chair or couch should not have a cushion pushing your head forward when you sit. Some older recliners used to have a round bulging pillow at the top of the chair that would constantly push your head forward and result in shoulder pain, headaches and breathing trouble. Avoid these types of recliners. It is important to change your seating arrangement daily by choosing to sit in a different chair or position on the couch each night. Human tendency is to keep everything the same; your favourite chair or your specific seat on the chesterfield, but my advice is to change it up. Every day pick a different place to sit. Your posture will love you for it.

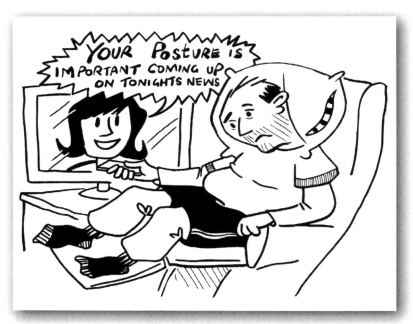

Notes

CHAPTER 2

RELIEF AND RESOLUTION FROM PAIN

*"Pain insists upon being attended to. God whispers to us
in our pleasures, speaks in our consciences, but shouts in
our pains. It is his megaphone to rouse a deaf world."*
– C.S. Lewis

In this chapter I want the tips I have listed here to really stand
out, so I have intentionally kept each tip clear and simple.
For those of you who want to know "why" the tips I mention
work so well, you can research the physiology online with 'Dr.
Google'. If your search does not automatically turn up our
blog, please click on our Blog and watch the television clips
where I attempt to quickly explain the 'why' behind all my recommendations. (Here is our blog page if you want to go right
to it: www.murphyhealthcentre.com/blog)

Also, please note that if you are experiencing painful symptoms, you should always have a proper examination of the problem
area by a professional (I am sure this is a legal requirement of me
to say this). Never do anything without professional supervision.

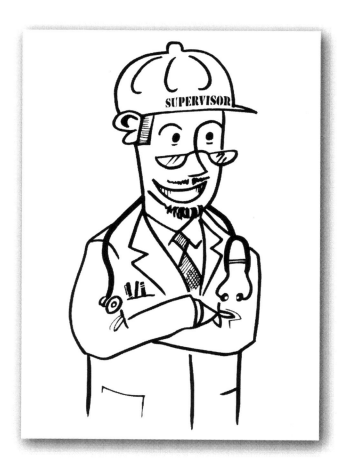

Shoulder pain

When you're experiencing shoulder pain that seems to have come on without an injury, it is usually because you have been keeping your arm bent too much. We bend our arm to hold our books, purse, baby, phone, briefcase, pressure washer, drill, hammer, newspaper, pen, in the car, at our desk, in our recliner, at the game...you get it. Over time, we will discover that our shoulder gets sore because of the imbalance of bent versus straightening. To help relieve the pain that is created by the imbalance, straighten your arm as often and as much as you can. To speed up your recovery, work your triceps (that's the muscle on the back of your arm) with a wall push-up. Improve your neck posture by keeping your chin up. This will aid the nerves to the shoulder. Walk and stand with your palms pointed forward to relax your shoulders.

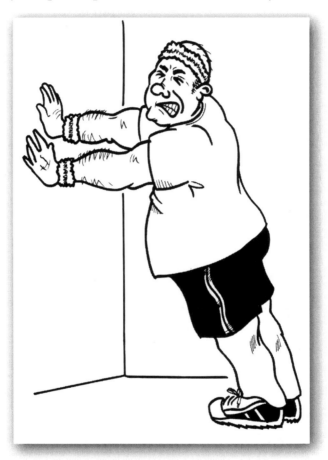

Doctor's tip... The one thing you need to be made aware of with respect to shoulder pain, is that both shoulders can be affected by organ problems. For example, when someone is experiencing a heart attack, often their left shoulder will be very sore and yet, the shoulder has nothing wrong with it? This is called "referred pain" and is due to the intricate arrangement of nerves that travel to the spine from the heart, as well as from the left shoulder. Both sets of nerves from the shoulder and the heart arrive at the same meeting point in the spine and so there is some overlap of signals which confuses the brain.

Liver and gall bladder problems are often causes of right shoulder pain, similar to the reasons we just saw above with your heart and left shoulder. It is important to rule these problems out when you are assessing your shoulder pain. Be sure to have a proper examination of your shoulder and spine by a Doctor of Chiropractic if the pain persists.

Knee pain

Knee pain usually means your body is dehydrated and acidic inside. Drink more spring, distilled or reverse osmotic bottled water. Add lemon to your water. When I say lemon, I mean a real, yellow lemon that you need to cut in half and literally squeeze the juice into your water. Some people try to use this tip and use lemon juice that is already prepared and bottled. This type of lemon juice will not balance the acid inside you because bottled lemon juice has additives that actually make you even more acidic! A real lemon will help stimulate your body to secrete more basic compounds into the blood and de-acidify your system.

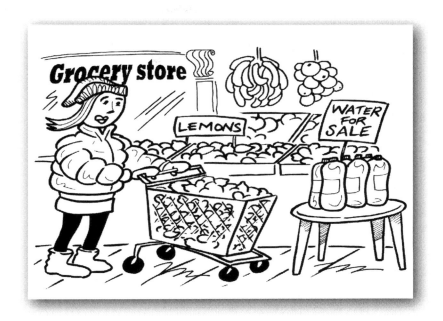

Doctor's tip... Many people have tests done when their knees are sore, either an MRI, X-ray or CT scan. I will caution you here because 9 times out of 10, these imaging studies will show wear and tear and arthritis in your knees. Please understand that while wear and tear and arthritis CAN cause knee pain, most people show signs of wear and tear and have *no* pain. This means we need to do a better job and find the real source of pain in your knees, rather than simply looking at these pictures. My recommendation is to stay with natural care of your knees for a while longer before considering surgery.

My Canadian thoughts on Surgery... In Canada, we consider surgery as an option WAY TOO MUCH!! I can tell you if we lived in the USA and we didn't have universal health insurance, surgery would not even be an option. Surgery is necessary only when your other option is a complete loss of the quality of your life. Mild pain on occasion in the knees is not something that should influence your quality of life, particularly if you can re-solve the problem with my tips here. The point is to trust the body you have been given at birth first.

If you are considering surgery ask yourself, *"If I don't have surgery will my other option be a wheel chair?"* If the answer to this question is a resounding, *"Yes"*, then you should consider the surgery. If you know you are giving up too easy, then wait! Remember that surgery is very invasive, no matter how skilled the surgeon. Once you have modified the inside of your body by cutting, cleaning, replacing and sewing, it will never be the same.

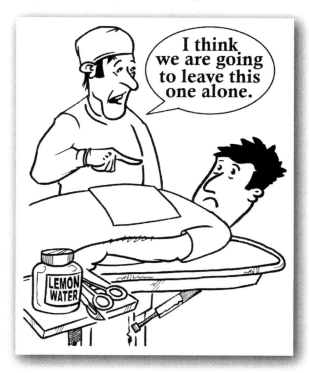

Arthritis pain

Pain from an arthritic joint can mean your body has become acidic inside, similar to knee pain mentioned already. Add a tablespoon of raw organic unpasteurized apple cider vinegar containing the mother (the mother is the most nutritious part of the apple cider vinegar and is very beneficial to digestion) to an 8-ounce glass of water per day. Drink 3 litres of water per day. Water is needed to keep your joints moving with ease.

You may be asking yourself, *"If I am too acidic doctor, why would I add acid like apple cider vinegar to my water?"* This is a good question. When you add the proper kind of apple cider vinegar that is all natural, raw and organic, with no citric acid added, you will cause your pancreas to release more bicarbonate, which will help the kidneys 'basify' your blood stream (or is it de-acidify? ...you get the point). You will achieve pain-free status when your blood stream becomes more natural.

Doctor's tip... The majority of people in North America are too acidic inside. Coffee, alcohol, heavy rich meals and gravies can all cause an imbalance creating an acidic internal environment. Normally the pH level of your insides is slightly basic with a pH of 7.4. If this balance shifts, it creates an abnormal, unhealthy, acidic internal environment and results in many of the problems we see clinically today.

Some of the effects of an acidic pH are:

- Burning joints
- Poor recovery after exercise
- Redness of the skin
- Pain
- Hastened digestion (food burns up faster and you usually have to run to the bathroom quickly after your meal)
- Accelerated arthritic changes

Gout pain

I mention a tip about gout pain here because it is one of the most painful types of arthritis. In order to buffer the pain of a gout attack, you should follow the recommendations above by adding natural apple cider vinegar to your diet and drinking 3 litres of quality water per day to flush the uric acid crystals out of your system. You can also add a supplement called URICA by a company called AOR during an outbreak as well, which seems to help recovery (AOR Supplements Canada contact information is at www.aor.ca).

> *Doctor's tip...* You can always tell when an outbreak of gout pain is coming because you will feel sharp pain in different joints from your neck to your back, from your hips to your knees. If you act quickly enough to re-establish your basic pH of 7.4 by following the recommendations for arthritis pain, your gout attack will be soothed before it starts.

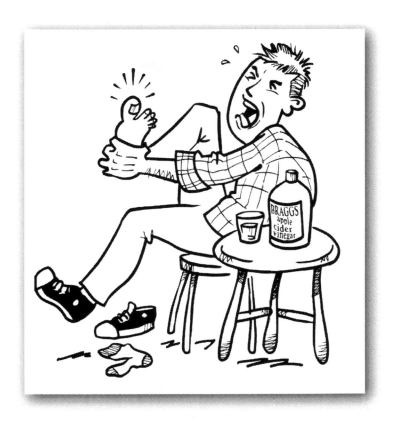

Head pain

Headaches are usually from poor posture in your neck and from having white stuff like flour and sugar in your diet. Follow our Daily Comfort Ideas mentioned in Chapter 1 and remove flour from your diet. Follow our posture tips and sitting tips (and basically everything I have mentioned already).

Doctor's tip... It is worth mentioning more about headaches here because I can't tell you how many times I have met a patient who says their healthcare provider told them that the headaches will never go away. People have been told they will suffer from headaches for the rest of their life. This destroys all hope of recovery and faith in the body to heal itself. Often times people are tested to confirm that there is no mass present or any other pressure-inducing cause. If a person isn't under a lot of stress or tension, usually a pain medication is recommended for their headaches. If the pain medication doesn't work, often a mood-altering drug is offered to help a person 'feel' better about the fact that they have 'incurable' headaches. This treatment method does not get to the source or cause of the problem and so it leaves me feeling uneasy as a doctor.

A person suffering from chronic headaches usually enters my clinic and asks for help with pain relief with only a glimmer of hope left inside them. Once we rule out the serious causes of head pain like masses and blood flow issues, we need to look at the spine.

The nerves that exit the spine at the base of the skull are almost always irritated when someone has head pain. By adjusting this area of the spine with chiropractic care, we have seen most people have complete resolution from head pain. *The spine is the secret.* Have your neck assessed by a chiropractor if you can't get relief of head pain.

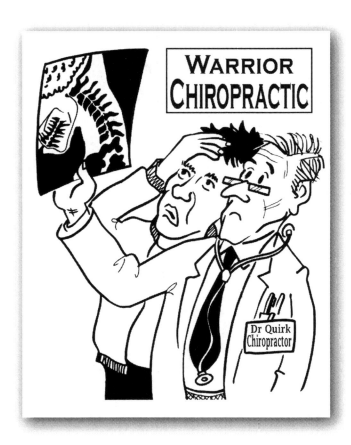

Stomach pain

People with chronic stomach pain are usually eating something that is overwhelming the digestive tract. The best advice is to cut out dairy and caffeine from your diet. To sooth an upset, gassy stomach, you can use peppermint Altoids (www.wrigley. com). You will have fresh breath, sleep better and have less pain if you follow this tip. Note here that some of my best friends are dairy farmers and they always hate when I tell people to cut out dairy. To those buddy's, I say, *sorry*. Rest assured that my simple recommendations will most likely not dent the dairy economy with the popularity of pizza, lasagne, chocolate milk and yoghurt. I simply believe that people with stomach pain will need to consider this tip for relief.

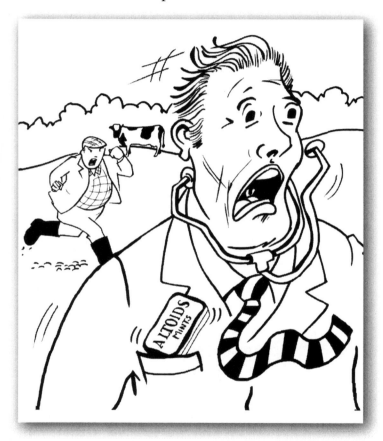

Doctor's tip... Introduced in 1780, Altoids mints were originally marketed to relieve stomach discomfort. The mints contain real peppermint which has been proven to be very helpful in relieving stomach pain. Peppermint flavour, on the other hand, will have no effect on stomach pain, so be sure to read the label.

Hip Pain (Sacroiliac joint)

Hip pain often shows up in people who have been sitting still for too long. When we sit the muscles of our legs and abdominals shorten. It is important to stretch the front of the hip by performing a lunge, alternating sides and holding each stretch. If this exercise is too difficult for you, you can place your shin on a rolling desk chair and lunge this way by simply rolling the supported leg backwards and holding it for a few seconds. Alternate this modified exercise from left to right as well. Note that the painful hip is not usually the problem hip - the pain-free hip is probably the provocative issue. A chiropractic assessment would confirm which hip is causing you the pain.

> *Doctor's tip...* Can you try something for me? Take your hands and slide them down your back to your tailbone. Feel the dimples at the base of your spine, or at least where they are supposed to be? When you say "hip" and I say "sacroiliac joint", we are usually talking about this same area. To be honest with you, the words 'hip' and 'sacroiliac' (SI for short) are not truly interchangeable, but it's ok for the purpose of this pain-relieving tip. Clinically speaking, your 'hip' is the top of your thigh where it enters your pelvis and the 'SI joints' are the

areas where your tail bone and pelvis meet (there, now you know something new and I can sleep at night).

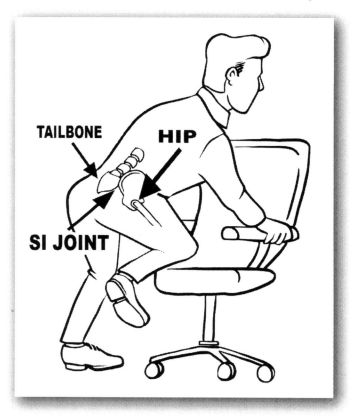

Back Pain

Back pain can be caused by so many things that the MOST IMPORTANT ADVICE I can give here is to have your spine assessed professionally by a Doctor of Chiropractic. The Chiropractor will be able to tell you why you are having pain and how to correct the problem that may be causing your pain.

Doctor's tip... The spine is too complex to be able to write one catch-all tip other than encouraging you to pursue a professional (I could write a whole book on this topic, actually!)

Notes

CHAPTER 3

RELIEF FROM MENTAL PAIN

*"Out of pain and problems have come the sweetest
songs, and the most gripping stories."*
– BILLY GRAHAM

If you have ever experienced a fogginess, a heaviness or a fullness in your head, then you have experienced what I like to call *brain noise*. You will know if you have experienced brain noise when all you want is for someone to hold your head for a few moments to give you relief. Besides physical pain, often the worst pain we can imagine is deep within our brain. Let's take a look at the more common causes of brain noise and the healthiest tips to improve on it.

Ups and Downs

When you notice your day is filled with mood swings, you are most likely suffering from the 'ups and downs' of a manic depressive type of brain noise. You can take a B complex vitamin daily all year and vitamin D3 in the Winter to help. You should also get sunshine at least 1/2 hour per day on top of your head and on your face. When the sun hits your face and head, it signals your body to produce more vitamin D. This vitamin helps stabilize your moods. Exercise for 1/2 hour per day to allow you to group your thoughts and avoid distractions. Pray and read for your spirit.

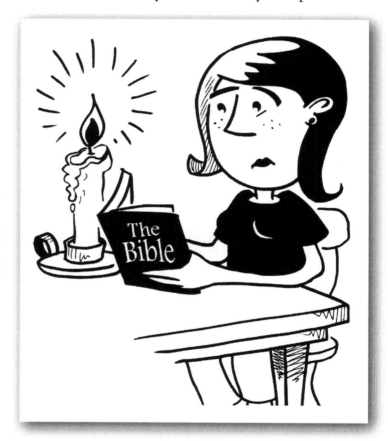

Depression
A heaviness causing a low mood is a quiet and sullen brain noise. If this occurs, you should follow vitamin advice for the

ups and downs and take a few other steps. You should cut out daily alcohol from your diet and lower coffee intake to 2 cups before noon. Change the focus from your daily needs and focus on the needs of everyone around you (sometimes I have to say this a few times to help it break through the brain noise). When you help others the hormone balance shifts deep inside you and you will feel a lift to your mood and spirit.

Start your day by waking up and asking God, *"Who can I help today?"* He will always provide you an answer to this question.

Anguish

Similar to the brain noise of the depressed, anguish is a mood that leaves a person feeling unmotivated to change. People who are experiencing this brain noise will have a very difficult time getting motivated to even begin to change. Take the advice above and do a good deed daily. Get addicted to doing good for others. The hormones dopamine, serotonin and oxytocin will be released inside you when you do good deeds and this will help you shake off the blues and discouragement.

Doctor's tip... Anguish often follows long term depression. When you have been depressed for a long time, the bad 'fight or flight' hormones like adrenaline, norepinephrine and cortisol will be too high in your system. These hormones change how you think and keep you stuck in fear. Excess fear leads to a complete loss of motivation and a feeling of an overwhelmed, sorrowful standstill. It is this cycle we want to change.

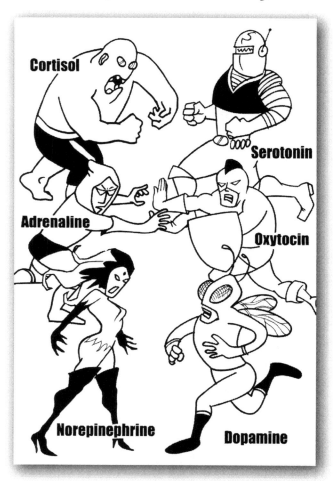

Anxiety

Brain noise associated with anxiety feels busy, rapid, loud, and restless. You can calm the brain noise of anxiety first by speaking with more respect to yourself. Follow the advice already mentioned in each section to help stabilize your mood. Anxiety is often the result of feeling nervous because of something that may happen in the future, where worry is about something that has happened in the past. Both feelings do not belong inside a healthy person. To combat the brain noise of anxiety, practice staying in the moment. Be present with loved ones and don't let your mind wander.

Biblically, God says He did not give you a spirit of fear, but of sound mind and spirit. Trust in the way you are created, worry less and fret not.

Doctor's tip... It is important to understand the difference between life-saving stress hormones and the positive hormones that can help you stabilize your life. When you were created, you were given hormones that are motivating chemicals that cause you to respond in specific ways when they are secreted into your blood.

The top three stress hormones that present themselves are: adrenaline, norepinephrine and cortisol. Picture a bear attacking you and you running like an Olympic sprinter to get away. In the case of emergency, adrenaline is released to give you a surge of energy and power. Under this stress, after a few moments, norepinephrine kicks in to help you maintain your emergency response until you arrive at safety. Finally, if the stress does not subside and it becomes chronic, cortisol kicks in to keep you running from danger.

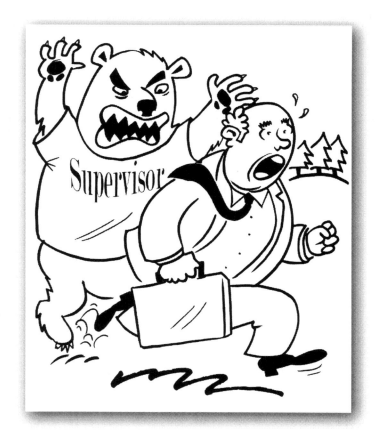

In modern times, we aren't usually fighting off bear attacks but it is possible that you are fighting off the stress from potential lay-offs, a sick loved one or even financial distress. These are every day stressors that we cannot run from so they often become chronic. Once chronic, an imbalance of stress hormones occurs inside resulting in depression, a poor immune system, high blood pressure, and memory loss, to name a few.

Fortunately, there are positive hormones that will help combat the effects of the bad, stress hormones, they are: dopamine, serotonin and oxytocin. You can create and control scenarios in your life where each of these good hormones will be secreted into your blood stream and bring about relief from chronic stress. Dopamine is released when you experience a 'high' from intense exercise. It is the hormone that creates the feeling of reward inside you. Serotonin is a hormone that is secreted when we feel proud of something and we are acknowledged publicly amongst our family and friends. Serotonin combats the effects of stress because it is the hormone that makes us feel 'pride' with our accomplishments. Serotonin is also released when we see others acknowledged for their accomplishments as well; think of the feeling you get when your spouse or children are honoured in public at an award show. The third hormone, Oxytocin, is the most powerful hormone of the three mentioned here because it is the hormone that gives us the 'warm fuzzy feeling' when we come into physical contact with someone we love. Hugs, handshakes, witnessing a good deed, and doing a good deed, all result in an Oxytocin surge. These three good hormones are essential to helping us combat the effects of chronic stress in our life. Keeping these hormones elevated in your system simply requires exercise, honouring others and loving the people around you.

Sleeplessness

While panic, chronic stress and caffeine can cause us to lose sleep, there is a natural bad habit most of us do daily that prevents our healthy sleep pattern. Most of us have lost our peaceful sleep routine that we had when we were children.

Remember when you would be winding down after supper as a child and you would have a light snack, a bath, read a story then quietly drift off to peaceful sleep? We need to do this as adults as well by creating a healthy sleep routine. Create a quieter, darker, calmer home environment starting one hour before bed. Watch only one hour of uplifting television per night. Read inspirational happy books and leave the murder mysteries and crime dramas for those people who want to stay awake. Program your brain every night with this routine and you will benefit with much better sleep.

Wakefulness

Sleeplessness and wakefulness sound like the same thing but these two types of brain noises are very different. Where sleeplessness is brain noise that prevents you from falling asleep, wakefulness is when you can fall asleep but keep waking up.

If you can get to sleep but you keep waking up in the early hours of morning, like 2, 3, 4am, then you can administer a change. Starting tomorrow get up as soon as you wake up any time after midnight, and reset the rhythm of the wakefulness and sleep cycle. For example, if you wake up at 3:30am, GET UP! I know it seems tough but it truly works. When you get up, you will reset your sleep cycle and sleep peacefully within a day or two.

Another cause of wakefulness is alcohol. Cut alcohol out of your diet and don't depend on its drowsiness effects. Alcohol becomes a stimulant when it is metabolized in the body causing you to wake up all throughout the night, leaving you exhausted all day. Enjoy an herbal tea after dinner instead of a glass of wine.

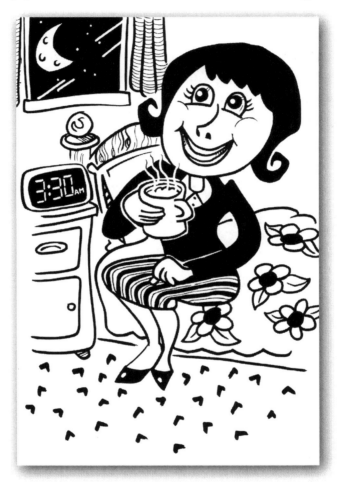

Forgetfulness
The brain noise of forgetfulness is a loud, buzzing, distracted panic. If you are experiencing memory issues, follow all the

advice above and purchase a journal to record your thoughts, appointments and daily routines. Be sure to add a B complex vitamin to your diet if you drink alcohol. Give yourself grace when you forget and avoid panicking when you do. Avoid distractions and speak slower. You will notice in time that you will become less forgetful when you allow yourself to forget some unnecessary daily tasks. Limit your daily requirements to simple, straightforward procedures. Plan out each day with the top three things you NEED to do and ignore the rest.

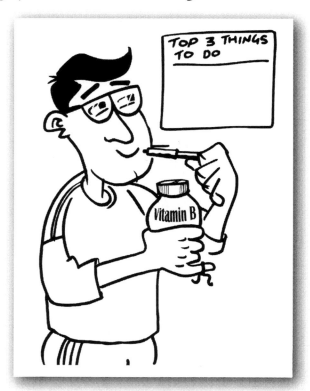

Doctor's tip... All the mental pain described here can be helped if we learn that something bigger than us is in control. We often experience brain noise when we are trying to control EVERYTHING. I believe in God and His word that tells me I have nothing to fear; He will provide everything I need.

Psalm 23 is often read to people at funerals or in Church on Sundays. If you don't have a Bible nor go to church, I am sure you could recite the first line of this Psalm with me from memory which states, *"The Lord is my provider, I have everything I need."* (You may know this line better from a different translation that states, "The Lord is my Shepherd, I shall not want", but the meaning is the same). God is in control, and when we believe this, we can shut off the brain noise and sleep peacefully. When we focus on the fact that we are put on this Earth as perfect creations to do good and to help others, we will see our worry, fear, anxiety, depression and panic disappear.

Notes

CHAPTER 4

SUPPORT FOR A HEALTHIER YOU

"You can't have a healthy civilization without healthy soil. You can't have junk food and have healthy people."
— JOEL SALATIN

As I mentioned earlier in the book, please always seek the advice of a qualified healthcare professional before trying any of the health tips I mention. Sometimes ignoring a proper exam will lead to dire consequences that could have been prevented. Please enjoy the tips in this section but understand the descriptions of organ problems here are not extensive nor complete and a proper exam is always necessary for proper diagnosis and treatment.

Let's imagine you are not experiencing any pain or discomfort but you notice a strange patch of dry skin, or maybe you notice dark circles and bags under your eyes. What happens if you have been told you are not digesting your food very well and this is why you are experiencing gas and bloating? How do you support your body to ensure that you will see improvement in how your systems function? This is what this section is all about; support for a healthier you.

Supporting your organ systems is sometimes a daunting task. We often don't understand what is causing the real problems we are experiencing because without pain, we don't always know where to begin. Your organs are all told what to do by your brain and nervous system. A proper spinal exam by a Doctor of Chiropractic will help you discover if there is a problem between the brain and your organs. This is important to rule out first.

Besides a spinal problem that may be causing your organ system issue, there may be an issue with the 'cleanliness' of your organ systems. If you have been consuming foods that have an endless shelf life or if you have been overwhelming your system with sugar, white flour, food colourings and chemicals, you will *definitely* want to purify your body by using some of these healthy tips.

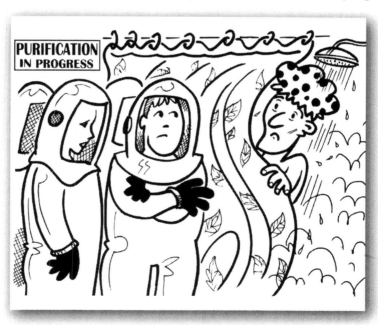

Liver support

To help purify your liver, add *real* lemon juice from a *real* lemon to 3 litres of water per day and consume. This helps sooth your liver. Your liver may be struggling if you have:

- Patches of psoriasis
- Mild discomfort under the last rib on your right side
- Right shoulder pain
- Yellowed skin or eyes
- Hormonal issues like 'menopause' or 'PMS'

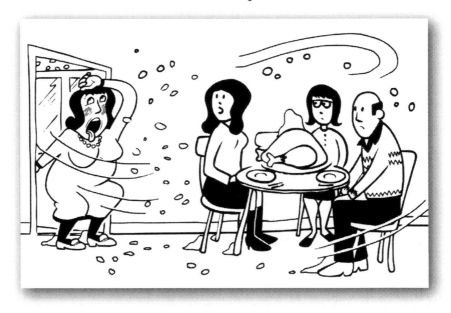

Bladder support

To help purify your bladder, add cranberry tablets to your diet in place of cranberry juice. Concentrated cranberry tablets are better than juice because the juice is full of sugar. Your bladder may be struggling if you have:

- Urine that smells bad
- Pain on urination
- Bed wetting issues
- Groin pain or lower abdominal pain
- Frequency or urgency of urination
- Infections that keep coming back

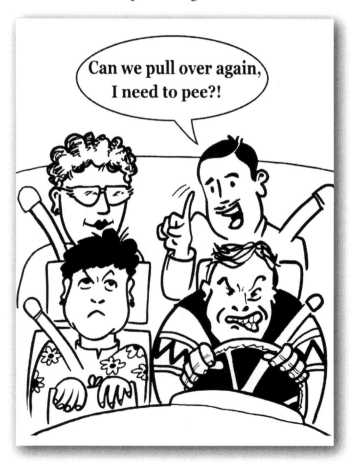

Kidney support

To help purify your kidneys, you can increase water intake as mentioned above, adding lemon like in the liver support section. Remove processed foods and eat REAL food from animals and plants only. You can add a tablespoon of baking soda to 8 ounces of water periodically to sooth hardworking kidneys. Kidneys work hard to establish a healthy pH in the body. The kidneys alone produce about two hundred and fifty grams (about half a pound) of bicarbonate per day in an attempt to neutralize acid in the body. Your kidneys could be struggling if you have:

- Upper mid back pain
- Dark circles under your eyes
- Blood pressure issues

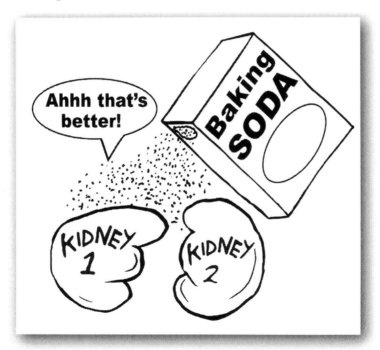

Heart support

To help purify your heart muscle, walk every day to the point where you break a sweat. If you complete your exercise and you have not begun to sweat, you did NOT exercise with enough intensity. Your heart is a muscle that benefits from exercise, water and healthy nutrition. Your heart may be struggling if you have:

- Tightness in your chest
- Difficulty catching your breath
- Left shoulder pain
- Jaw pain
- No noticeable symptoms at all (this is true in most cases of a struggling heart)

Doctor's tip... Chiropractic spinal restorative care of your upper and mid back has been demonstrated in research to benefit heart health. The nerves that travel from the brain to the heart exit the spine near the top of your back. If you have poor posture where your head is forward of your shoulders and you notice a hump forming on your upper back, please call a Doctor of Chiropractic to assess your spine. The chiropractic assessment may help you discover the cause of your struggling heart.

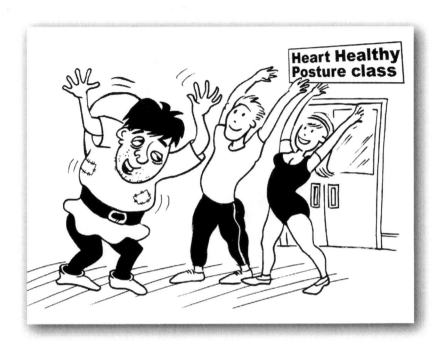

Lung support

To help purify your lungs you can cut out dairy from your diet to lower mucus, and add lemon to 3 litres of quality water and consume daily. Practice diaphragm breathing by inspiring through your nose WITHOUT making sniffing noises. Pull air in through your nose to your belly and expire slowly through your mouth with a relaxed jaw. The secret here is to be sure to pull air all the way into your belly and avoid breathing 'high' in your chest. Singers practice this skill all the time to be able to hold that BIG FINAL NOTE! Your lungs may be struggling if you have:

- Difficulty sleeping
- Sensitivity to very cold air
- A lot of phlegm production
- The need to clear your throat before you speak
- Frequent sinus infections

Doctor's tip... It is important here to outline what constitutes 'dairy-free' eating. Eating dairy-free means that you remove milk, cheese, yoghurt, butter, and cream from your diet in all forms. If it comes from the cow's udder, avoid it. You also need to remove dairy additives in foods that you eat. Often milk protein in the form of casein is added to flavourings to give a 'cream' taste to foods. You'll find casein listed on labels as: casein, caseinates, calcium caseinate, potassium caseinate and sodium caseinate. I have seen 'dairy-free' cheese with casein protein added, which essentially causes the same symptoms as if a person was drinking a glass of milk. The problem with the milk protein casein as an addictive is that it is very difficult to digest. Overall, casein is a protein that challenges your system and you should avoid it to support your health.

Stomach support

To help purify your stomach, eat food from plants and animals *only*. Food that lasts in a can, bag or on the shelf for longer than three days is not healthy for consumption. Follow the liver and kidney support already mentioned. Avoid stimulants like caffeine and alcohol in your diet as well as dairy, flour and sugar. You have the potential to heal your digestive tract by simply eating smarter. Your stomach may be struggling if you have:

- Alternating constipation and diarrhea
- Difficulty losing weight
- Bloating after meals
- Nausea and gas
- Pain

Doctor's tip... Some people tell me that they cannot eat real fruit or vegetables. They explain that eating some fruits or vegetables causes a digestive upset due to a reaction with their medication. I grow quite concerned when a pharmaceutical is preventing someone from eating naturally. To these people, I recommend discussing their medications with their Medical Doctor (their MD) and explain their desire to eat fruit, vegetables and other nutrients from the earth. There must be a need to change or alter any medication that prevents us from eating healthy.

Brain and nervous system support

To enhance the purity of your nervous system, you can have an assessment by a Doctor of Chiropractic. If you are a candidate for spinal care, please get on a proper spinal restoration program. Spinal adjustments nourish your brain because 90% of all nourishment to the brain comes from spinal movement only. We either move it or lose it and since you can't literally move your brain, you have been designed to move your spine instead.

Your brain is housed deep within your skull but it is also housed within an articulating spinal column with 24 moveable parts. Each one of these articulations need to move freely and properly. When an area of your spine has been damaged or misaligned, this leads to irritation of the nerves in these areas which can cause spinal damage. If you leave spinal damage uncorrected symptoms can occur.

Doctor's tip... My belief about chiropractic spinal restoration:

Chiropractors save lives by helping correct the spine
The spine improves with movement
The more we positively stimulate the spine and nervous system, the healthier it becomes (think about practicing and playing an instrument or sport, the more you practice the better you get)
The nervous system learns through stimulation
You are designed to heal from birth through your nervous system
When your nervous system is healthy, your body will be healthy
If your spine is breaking down it rarely causes pain
Spinal decay leads to a loss of function in your body
An exam by a Chiropractor is important

Posture support

To help purify your posture, walk every day for at least 30 minutes. Be sure to break a sweat and let your mind wander. Keep your chin up while you walk, look forward, swing your arms with your palms facing forward, relax your shoulders, breathe in through your nose and out your mouth, slowly and intentionally. Stand tall, know you are great and *smile*.

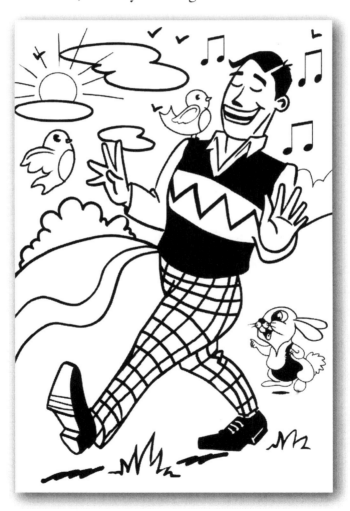

Muscle Support

To help purify your muscles, add water with lemon to your diet as mentioned already. Take a multivitamin to help ensure you have all the right building blocks for your muscles. Exercise regularly to break a sweat. Registered massage therapy is very helpful to address sore and aching muscles. Your muscles will do what they are told to do by the nervous system, so be sure to always have your spine assessed by a Chiropractor. If your nervous system is healthy, you have a greater potential to have healthier muscles that recover from injury with ease.

Skin Support

To help purify your skin please follow the water intake instructions above by drinking 3 litres of pure water a day, including lemon if you can. Understand that your skin is a window to the inside of your body. The health of your liver and digestive tract will dictate how your skin will look. Follow all organ support recommendations mentioned already to create the purest internal environment you can. Healthier organs will result in healthier skin.

> *Doctor's tip...* A skin disorder like psoriasis can be due to liver function trouble, make sure to support your liver. Eczema can be due to dehydration and you should follow rehydration recommendations noted above. Acne can be helped by helping your body digest better foods

and nutrients. The purer your insides, the purer your outside.

Hormone Support

To purify the secretion of hormones (I know I am really stretching the 'purify' in this sense), be sure to do good deeds, acknowledge people and honour people in your life. When you do these things, good hormones increase and bad stressful hormones decrease. Exercise to the point of sweating. Rehydrate and have your spine assessed by a Doctor of Chiropractic. Support your detoxifying organs like your liver, skin and kidneys by eating natural foods. Avoid meats that have been injected with synthetic hormones and tap water that does not filter out hormones.

> *Doctor's tip...* There are many studies being conducted on the rise of pharmaceuticals in our drinking water due to the number of people taking prescription and non-prescription medications and then urinating back into the ecosystem. Our current filtration systems do not remove these pharmaceuticals and pollutants thus allowing spillover from all pharmaceuticals into our water. Birth control pills, hormone replacement pills, phytoestrogens and waste from animals injected with hormones, all find their way into our drinking water. This is important to note for those of you struggling with an imbalance in your hormone production.

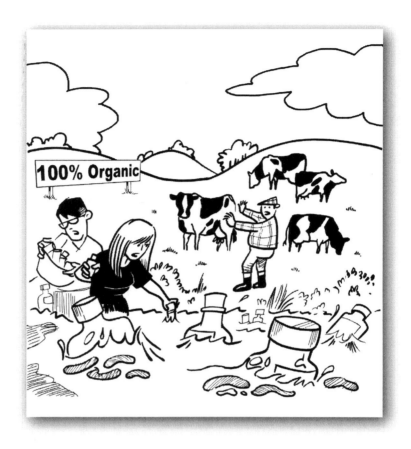

Notes

CHAPTER 5

WEIGHT LOSS AND TONING

"As for my diet, I try to eat lean, clean and healthy - nothing too surprising. And I avoid too much meat or dairy because they slow you down."
— BEAR GRYLLS

O ne of the most common questions I receive each year is, *"How do I lose weight?"* Other than cutting down the calories you eat and exercising more, some people still have trouble losing weight.

What I have found is that some people have enormous success in losing weight and others seem to get frustrated with their lack of success. Some people want to lose weight from their mid-section and others want to lose weight from their face. Some people base their success on toning their body, others base it on the number displayed on the scale. In this chapter I want to share the best tips I can give you with respect to your weight and how you can lose it quickly and tone up your body.

Achieve a Tighter, Flatter Stomach

When you have a chubbier than normal midsection, no matter how many abdominal crunches you perform, you need to change your approach. If you are searching for a tighter flatter stomach, you need to start by lengthening and tightening the abdominal muscles. You can flatten your stomach by performing planks as well as using hand held rollers for abdominal exercises. It is my belief that most people need to avoid crunches for their abdominal exercises because most people sit too much already. Crunches force you back into this sitting posture by shortening your stomach and hip muscles. Crunches tend to overstimulate short hip flexor muscles which results in hip pain, lower back pain and a chubbier midsection. This is obviously not your goal. We don't need any more exercise that puts us into a slumped forward posture than we already have at our desk, driving or watching television in our favourite chair.

Your goal is to flatten your stomach and so you should lengthen your abdominal muscles during exercise and keep them tight.

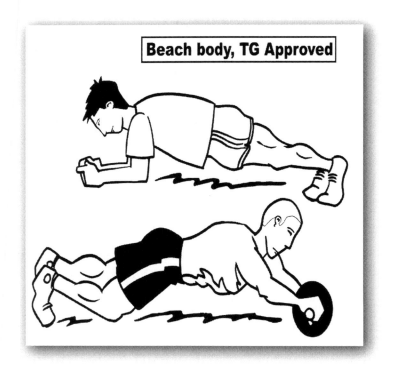

Beach body, TG Approved

Diet Modification to Deflate that Spare Tire

If you are doing the exercises I mentioned to flatten your stomach muscles and you are still not seeing great changes, then we need to look at some diet modification to help. The first step to deflate the spare tire around your waste is to drink less caffeine. Lowering coffee and other caffeinated beverages will lower the number of stimulants you intake in your diet. The purpose of eliminating the stimulants from your diet is to decrease cortisol in your blood stream. Following the healthy tip to flatten your stomach and removing coffee, tea, and caffeinated soda, will lower the stress on your system. Less system stress will lower cortisol levels in your blood stream and therefore decrease the fat deposition around your waist and hips.

Slim Down that Double Chin

One of the best ways to decrease the weight around your face is to remove carbonated drinks from your diet, like beer and soda. You should also remove flour and sugar from your diet. When you remove these things from your diet, you will experience less bloating which will be evident in your face.

Pack Away the Bags Under Your Eyes

Follow the kidney support ideas mentioned in chapter 4. Dark circles and puffiness under your eyes are usually due to over-worked kidneys. Rehydrate with quality water and drink 3 litres per day. Follow our healthy sleep recommendations and be sure to support your digestion as suggested.

Kick up a Sluggish Metabolism

When you feel like your metabolism is sluggish and you want it to kick up a notch, be sure to exercise your large thigh muscles. The best exercises to perform several times a week are the following:

- Squats, stairs, and box jumps for the athlete
- Walking, running, stairs, and hiking for the outdoor person
- Sit/stand from a chair for the everyday person

Working these muscle groups in your thighs communicates to your brain that you are choosing to work your body harder and your metabolism will change. You will burn more calories and see positive changes from exercise much more quickly.

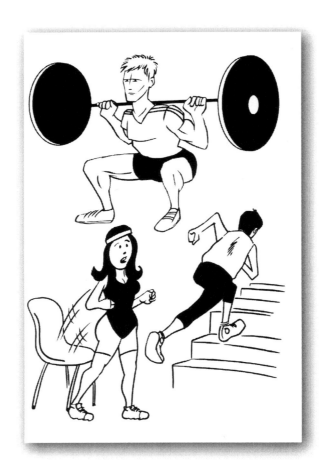

To Float the Bloat

To remove bloating after meals, avoid white flour, processed foods and sugar. Avoid carbonated beverages and only eat REAL food. Real food is food grown in the ground and meat from an animal. The healthiest food you can eat will rot after a few days if left sitting on the counter. If the food you want to eat does not rot, it will not break down easily in your body. Therefore, avoid potato chips, canned goods, food in bags, and food in boxes.

Doctor's tip... Remember you are beautiful. What you focus on will surely come to pass. You may tell yourself many times a day that you are too fat! Stop! Tell yourself that you are beautiful and that you are getting more toned. Tell yourself you are taking the appropriate steps to lose weight and you are looking really good! Say, *"I am on my way! I am in great shape! I can do this!"* You will be amazed at how quickly you will tone up when you speak to yourself with kindness and love. Trust me.

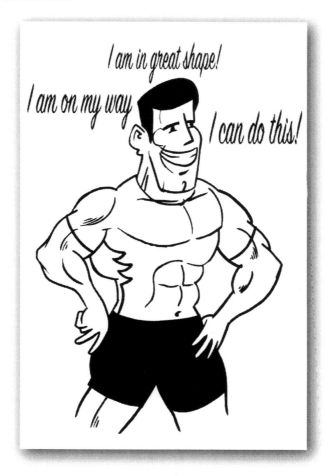

Notes

CHAPTER 6

HEALTHY LIVING THROUGH RELATIONSHIPS

*"I believe that the greatest gift you can give your
family and the World is a healthy you."*
— Joyce Meyer

Health is an above-down inside-out process. Your pursuit of better health spreads out into everyone and everything around you. Leading by example is key to helping people achieve greatness. Your physical health, the health of your family, a healthy workplace, your healthy choices at the fitness centre and your spiritual health are all part of achieving a better life. In this chapter I discuss the best tips for helping you lead by example.

Different relationships have a different priority in your life. You should focus on your relationships in the following order: God first, then spouse, then children, then colleagues, then everyone else. For the purpose of this section, I will focus on the groups you interact with directly from top-down, ending with a short blurb about fitness health. I added fitness health here because achieving better fitness health is directly linked to improving your core relationships.

Spirit Health

I would be amiss if I didn't talk about spirit health in a book about healing tips. Personally, I believe that your spiritual health is the most important part of proper healing and living well. Spirit health is intricately intertwined with your belief system. By this I mean you will act out what you believe in your life. If you believe there is a power greater than yourself, you will live to discover more about that power. If you feel like YOU are 'all there is' in this life, you will most likely have difficulty believing in a Greater Power and you can probably skip this section. If you find you fit into the latter category, I still hope you read on and keep an open mind.

My tips to help you believe and live each day healthy and whole:

Find a Bible that is easy to read. There are loads of translations out there and I have discovered that one reason people don't read their Bible is because they don't understand it. Choose a New Century Version or New Language Translation. Both are very easy to read and understand.

Pick a time to read your Bible each day. I like reading in the morning when my house is quiet. Read from the beginning or choose to start anywhere you like when you read your Bible. Some people like to start in the New Testament (which is near the back starting with the book of Matthew) and others will start on page one, chapter one, verse one of Genesis (the first book of the Bible). It doesn't matter where you start, just start.

You can download an app that helps you go through the Bible by using devotional writings that lead you through scripture verses. This is a great way to learn the Bible and what it means.

I recommend you find a good Bible-based Church to help you grow spiritually. Remember, God wants a relationship with you, not necessarily a religion. But it is nice to go to Church and sing and worship Him. There is something special about getting together with like-minded individuals and celebrating the Lord.

Live out what you learn in the Bible *every day*. When you are ready, pray for forgiveness of any wrongs that you feel need to be lifted off your spirit.

Ask God to come into your life by simply saying out loud, *"God, please come into my life and find ways to connect with me as I search for you."* He'll find you when you ask Him to. He is always pursuing you.

Be prepared to be amazed at your life and the relationship you will develop with God.

Don't over-think the steps you take to discover more about God.

Give yourself some grace while you learn.

Believe you can change for the better.

Remember the simplest people have found a relationship with God to be the most satisfying, peace-inducing, loving relationship of their lives (I'm excited for you!)

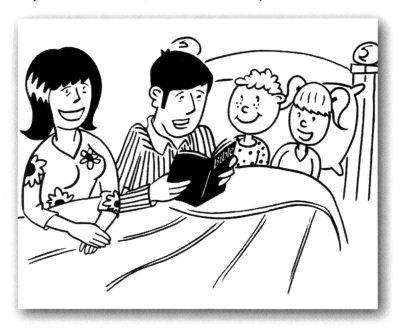

Spouse Health

Next to God, your spouse is the most important person in your life. When you prioritize your spouse, you will be blessed and so will they. Here are some tips to keep that flame burning bright:

When you arrive home, search out and hug your spouse first before everyone else.

Smile when you see your spouse no matter how you are feeling.

When your spouse asks you how your day was, always answer that it was good. Your spouse is not asking you about your day to hear you unload every bad or irritating occurrence from the day (even though they won't tell you that to your face).

Always stand by your spouse and demonstrate your love every day.

Honour your spouse both when they are around, and when they are not.

Always be more kind to your spouse than anyone else.

Defend your spouse FIRST.

When disagreements arise, remember you are fighting FOR your spouse, not WITH your spouse.

Protect your spouse by praying for them all the time.

Search out different ways to help your spouse every day.

When going to sleep, be sure you tell your spouse what you love about them. Be specific and sincere.

Share what you love about your children with your spouse.

Pray together.

Children's Health

After your spouse comes your children. Your children need to see and learn that your spouse comes first before their needs are met. In order to see your children have an amazing life, follow some of these tried and tested tips:

Tell your children why you love them every day. Be specific. Pack lunches together for school and prepare meals together.

Remove fear from their lives by being fearless yourself.

Teach them to go after their goals, by making sure you go after *your* goals.

Teach your children good eating habits by having good eating habits of your own.

Be present and become a good listener. Your children will begin to open up about their lives when you make yourself available.

Dream together.

Work Health

When you work in an office or where other people are present, remember these important tips to be sure you end your day feeling positive and healthy.

Go into work the same way an actor walks on stage. Remember, you are performing from the time you enter work to the time you go home.

Choose your words carefully and speak with respect to your co-workers and supervisor.

Work just as hard in front of people as on your own.

Remember, promotions come from God, not from your boss. Work hard, do your best work and know that God sees your effort.

Set clear boundaries for where work ends and where your personal life begins.

Keep your online life (Facebook, Instagram, Twitter and other social media platforms) private.

When you arrive home, leave every bad encounter outside before you enter your house.

Keep your home life sacred.

Be honest, always.

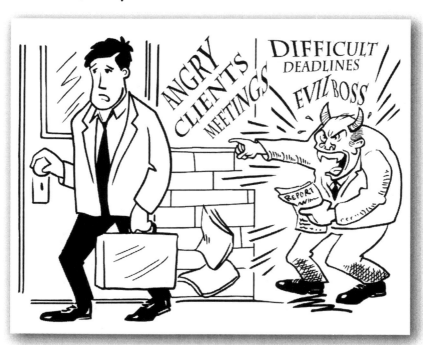

Fitness Health

Training for life is physical, mental, social and spiritual. If you want the best relationships in your life, you need to train hard physically. Good relationships require hard work so you need to be at your physical best. Here are key fitness tips to help you stay at the top of your game:

Set goals to stay motivated.

Motivation is easiest when you publicly declare your goals.

Commit yourself to a fitness class.

Hire a trainer. Fitness is most effective when you are able to think less and act more.

Workouts should be short, intense, fun and challenging.

Plan for an intense 30-45 minutes per workout.

Don't cut corners.

Celebrate your achievements!

Doctor's tip... My favourite type of exercise is done in a boutique setting; with other people in a class with fun music. A good class has a spirited trainer who has prepared the class ahead of time. The best classes only last 45 minutes maximum. When you exercise in this type of setting, you will see great changes in yourself. You will discover what you can truly accomplish all while having fun. When your fitness reaches a decent level, you will have plenty of energy to be at your best in all areas of your life, including all your relationships.

Notes

CHAPTER 7

THE DOCTOR IS IN!

"The doctor of the future will give no medicine but will interest his patients in the care of the human frame, in diet and the cause and prevention of disease."
– THOMAS EDISON

In practice, I care for the needs of people who are often in a lot of distress and pain. Over the years there have been specific questions and concerns that have come up more frequently than others. I would like to use this final chapter to outline and discuss some of the more common topics that have come up in daily conversation. I hope to help you gain a greater insight into some very complex topics to bring more certainty and comfort to your life. I will discuss the meaning behind some common symptoms, give you an overview of the flu season myth, and outline two fascinating healing methods to finish the chapter.

Symptoms are important

When you experience symptoms of any kind, don't suppress the symptoms, *support* them. Symptoms keep you alive. Fever, vomiting, pain, numbness, increased blood pressure, fatigue and sleeplessness are all important. As a healthcare provider, I want to teach you how to support yourself during these times of symptom awareness, so you will have less fear, less stress, and more understanding of how your body works.

Pain

You need to feel pain to know your limits. For example, let's say you choose to rake your lawn for 4 hours and you notice you are sore 2-3 days later. This teaches you that raking for 4 hours after not raking all summer may be a bad idea. Journal that thought and learn the lesson for next time. The symptom of pain in this example helps you to discover your limits.

Pain can be caused by many things, including:

- Overuse
- Dehydration
- Eating nightshade vegetables (Tomatoes, potatoes and bell peppers)
- Trauma
- Mental disturbances

Pain is usually the last symptom to show up when a problem persists for too long. Your brain interprets physical pain from the body the same as mental pain from your mind. The pain of a loss or death is as real to the brain as breaking your arm.

The mental processing is very similar. It's all pain and it all hurts.

> *Doctor's tip...* Celebrate pain! Pain means you are still alive and your nervous system is working properly. Learn from the pain and be honest with yourself. Change what needs to be changed and seek help if you need it. Chiropractors basically specialize in pain because we specialize in spinal health, the brain and nervous system. We are experts at helping you discover where the pain may be coming from and how to solve the issue naturally. *Don't ignore pain that won't go away.*

Numbness

Numbness is an indication that your nervous system is working properly and yet something is irritating a nerve. Numbness can be a 'pins and needles' sensation or a complete loss of feeling in a specific area of your body.

> *Doctor's tip...* When you feel numbness, understand that a nerve is involved. If you notice pins and needles from simply sitting on your leg for too long or leaning awkwardly on your arm, then I suggest you change position. On a more serious note, if you feel like a part of your body has been frozen by anaesthetic but it hasn't, seek professional help. Sometimes a complete lack of sensation can be quite severe and lead to serious complications. Don't ignore numbness that doesn't improve with movement.

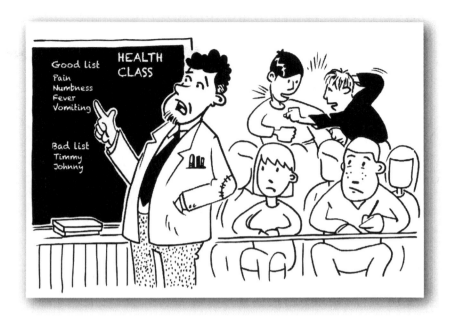

Vomiting

When you vomit, your body is telling you that it does not like what you are ingesting. If the food you eat is full of toxic bacteria, your body wants to get it out of you. Imagine you ate something poisonous and you started to vomit. In that moment, your brain is trying to save your life. Now let's say you run to the medicine cabinet and take some drug to shut down your ability to feel nauseous or your ability to vomit. Now that poison is allowed to stay inside you because you prevented your body from expelling it.

> *Doctor's tip...* It's always healthier to let your body expel the poison through vomiting than to let the poison stay inside your stomach and enter your bloodstream. Trust

your body, it knows best. If you have excessive vomiting, be sure to let your Chiropractor know. Never ignore vomiting if it persists.

Fever

Most of us have grown up thinking that any body temperature above normal is serious (normal body temperature is 37 degrees Celsius or 98.6 degrees Fahrenheit). *This is not true!* When your body increases temperature, it is fighting something and usually doing a great job. Increased temperature is one of the most effective ways your body can fight infection. Your body needs fever to protect you. Viruses, bacteria and parasites hate fevers because high fevers kill these bugs.

> *Doctor's tip...* Don't fear your fever. Monitor the fever and trust your body. Avoid medications that artificially prevent fevers. Use cold compresses to lower high fevers and communicate with your Chiropractor. Remember, if you take a drug to decrease pain it will also artificially decrease your body temperature preventing your body from producing a proper fever.

Increased Blood Pressure

Your heart will increase pressure for many reasons. One of the most common reasons your blood pressure increases is when you are anxious and feeling panic. Most of the time your blood pressure will increase to prepare you for a stressful 'fight or flight' situation. The problem is, sometimes stress is chronic and your blood pressure is forced to stay elevated for too long.

> *Doctor's tip...* If you are experiencing elevated blood pressure from chronic stress (work, relationships, personal etc.) then deal with the true problem before you take medication. Change your career, work on the problem relationship, or seek professional counselling. Mental issues can create physical outcomes in your body and blood pressure elevation is one of the most common.

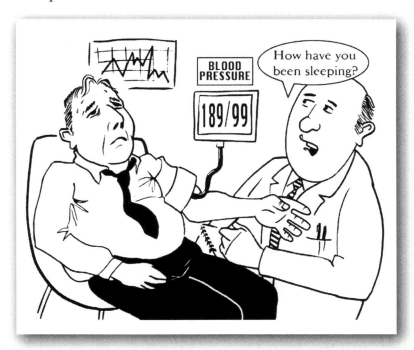

Fatigue

One of the most common causes of fatigue is chronic stress. Many people today are experiencing fatigue because they are working too hard with limited holidays, alongside unhappy people, in a job that does not fulfil them, under restrictive deadlines, with overwhelming expectations. Similar to increased blood pressure, fatigue will set in when you have not managed chronic stress very well.

> *Doctor's tip...* You can change! You are in control of your life and you have the power to change careers. You are not guaranteed tomorrow so you need to take the steps to change today. You should be working at something that fulfils your life purpose. You have talents and God-given skills that need to be exercised to change the world outside you as well as the world inside you. When you are doing what you were put on this Earth to do, you will feel fulfilled, happy and refreshed every day. Don't be scared to change - your life depends on it.

Sleeplessness

I have experienced sleeplessness myself for most of my life. There is a positive side and a negative side to this symptom. The positive sleeplessness is when someone is so excited to do something great that they can hardly wait until morning. That is GOOD sleeplessness and that is usually me.

The negative sleeplessness is related to anxiety and worry. If your sleeplessness is due to anxiety and worry, it can mean that your faith has grown weak. Biblically, God tells us to trust in Him and He will give us rest. If we believe this, we will sleep well. If we do not believe or trust that God will take care of us, we will probably toss and turn all night, worrying about how to control the outcomes ourselves.

Doctor's tip... Any time you can't sleep you need to assess the cause. Trust God. Read your Bible and believe what it says. If you struggle with your belief, pray that God will help you achieve peace in your life, and He will. Believe.

The Flu Season Myth

There is no such thing as 'flu season'. There is no season where the flu comes alive and no season where flu is hiding. Viruses don't take vacations nor do they hide. Every virus is present all year, as are you.

So why do we get sick more frequently at certain times of the year? We get sick because we become more vulnerable due to our diet and our bad habits. We become more vulnerable to viruses, bacteria, fungus and parasites when we are worn out and run down. At these times, we are usually lacking necessary vitamins, rest, immunity and sunshine.

Clinically, we can be sure a person will have a difficult time with illness between late September until early April because:

- We are eating more sugar (Halloween, Christmas, Easter)
- We are drinking more alcohol and coffee

- We are breathing less fresh air
- We are not in the sun
- We are cold and chilled more frequently
- We are not 'grounding' ourselves as much (I'll explain what grounding is)
- We are not exercising
- We are not purging the dampness from our lungs (I'll explain this one too)

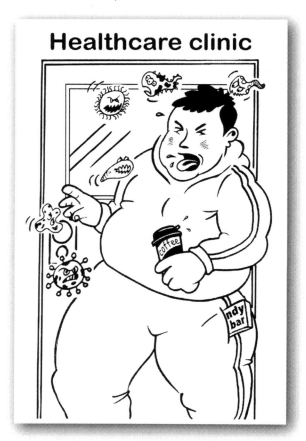

We become more vulnerable to viruses and bacteria on doorknobs, airborne bugs, restaurant food, and everywhere else during these vulnerable months mentioned above. If you support yourself using the tips I have suggested throughout this book, you will be stronger and healthier more often. You will be able to fight the flu and any other bug that tries to knock you down. You have an immune system that has served you for your whole life, long before any flu shot came into the picture.

> *Doctor's tip...* The commercials I hear during the months of September and October about the flu and the flu shot make me more nauseous than the flu itself. The reason these commercials upset me so, is because they attempt to blame innocent children as the evil 'carriers' of the flu and we need to protect ourselves from them!

If you learn nothing more from this section than this, please note: *You and I get infected with every single 'bug' every single day.* We are no better than any innocent child. The reason we do not get sick every single day is because God created you and I with an amazing immune system that works perfectly when we support ourselves properly. And guess what, God didn't forget to give the beautiful children an immune system either. Children have awesome immunity too, and the way their immunity grows is through fighting the bugs. Let's leave the children alone and let them grow the way they were supposed to grow.

I could write an entire book on the abuse of pharmaceutical companies on the civilized nations of the World through media, falsehoods and fear tactics, but I better step off my soapbox and stay civil for the positive purposes of this book (deep breath in and ahhhhh... there I feel better).

Grounding yourself

I mentioned grounding as a method to keep ourselves healthy during the vulnerable months of September to April. I would like to explain this simple yet effective concept.

We are carrying electronics and powered devices with us every day. Researchers are now discovering the need to 'ground' ourselves to remove the static electricity from our bodies. Humans have insulated themselves from contact with the earth by wearing synthetic soled shoes and living in homes that elevate the body above the earth. Consequently, humans are no longer naturally grounded. Now the body becomes charged with static electricity which creates unnatural, weak electric currents in the body. This is worse in the Winter.

Have you ever noticed how in the Winter when you reach out to shake someone's hand, just as you get close, an electric arc crosses from your fingers to the unsuspecting victim and *ZAP*, you shock them? Do you ever wonder why this happens more in the Winter than the Summer months? The answer is that you are building up more electricity during the dry Winter months and so you need to be 'grounded'. Just like an open circuit on a farmer's electric fence, you become the ground for someone else when you feel the shock.

The way to stop this annoying and sometimes painful problem is to 'ground' yourself by getting your feet on the ground, uninsulated by the rubber soles of your shoes and boots. Less insulation between your body and the ground will help you to remove the excess electricity from your body.

In order to stay healthy throughout the Winter, it is essential to rid yourself of the static electricity and get outside and ground yourself. This is another important reason to exercise outside during the Winter months.

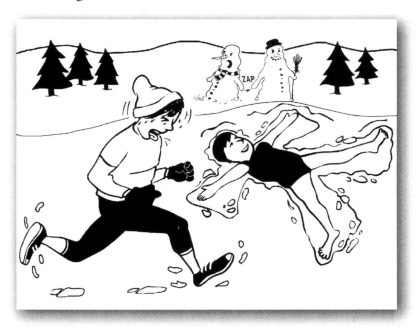

Purge the Dampness

Another important Winter exercise is to purge the dampness from your body. If you are not exercising much, you probably don't exercise at all during the Winter. If you sit sedentary from day to day, consuming dairy foods and other phlegm producing food sources, I can guarantee that you are experiencing an 'attack of dampness' according to the Chinese medicine experts.

When your lungs and sinuses fill up with moisture that sits stagnate in your body, you will most certainly develop an irritating cough or sinus issue at some point throughout the year, especially in the Winter. It is important to purge this dampness.

To purge the dampness, you need to increase your blood flow, breathing and heart rate. If you are thinking, *"Wow, that sounds like he is talking about exercise."* You are right!

Earlier in the book I mention that the proper way to exercise is to exercise enough to create sweat. If you are exercising to the point where you are breathing harder and you are sweating, you will begin to notice that your nose will run and you may have to clear your throat more frequently by coughing. This is how your body purges the dampness. Let your nose run to drain your sinuses and cough as much as you need to rid the phlegm from your lungs. Regular exercise on a daily basis in the Winter is essential to prevent illness and infections because it allows your body to rid itself of excess dampness.

Notes

EPILOGUE

This book has been a labour of love for me. It has been a book that has been in various stages of writing for 20 years. As I reread the different chapters and edit the content, I can see that there will be revisions and updates as my experience grows.

I have intentionally kept the science to a minimum as well as the language of the text clear and simple. I don't need to *wow* you with fancy words, nor bore you with all the scientific research. I simply want a book that you can read and enjoy.

I started out with the intention to make the book simple, short, funny and clear. I didn't want to bog you down with research paper summaries and references that you can easily find online yourself.

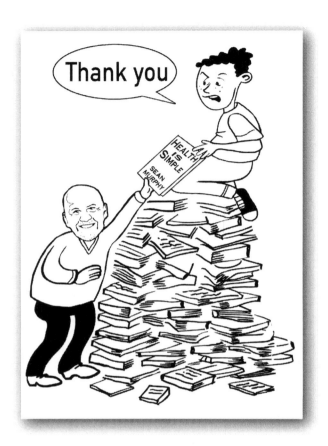

This book is for *real* people experiencing *real* problems. The tips I share are for *you*. Perhaps you will share this book with a friend. Perhaps you will even try some of the tips mentioned here for yourself. Whatever it is, you can be certain that there will be more coming from Dr. Sean Murphy in the future! (I always hate when someone talks about themselves in the third person but wanted to give it a try).

So, from me to you, I hope you enjoyed the simplicity of it all. Thank you for reading.

GENERAL HEALTH SUMMARY

Now to finish in general terms, I want to summarize some of the most common recommendations I make to everyone I know:

Get your spine assessed by a trained Doctor of Chiropractic. This helps you correct the real problems from the inside out.

Ice at night, warm in morning. When you are using temperature to help with pain and function, warm up for your day and cool down at night. Never do the opposite or you will be sorry the next day. Many people use a heating pad for pain at night before bed, but notice in the morning that the pain and stiffness is much worse. Always cool down a problem area at night and warm up in the morning. Think of your day like a sport you play.

Remove foods like white potatoes, flour and sugar for 30 days and see if your pain decreases and your health improves.

Change where you sit every night. Habits cause problems if they are unhealthy. One of the worst unhealthy habits is to sit the same way, in the same chair, for the same length of time, every day. Change is good.

Change your pillow. This seems simple but pillows only last about 6 months. Invest in great pillows and use the old ones for throw pillows (learn how to sew).

Change your chair. Similar to your pillow, change the chair you sit on at work. In an office setting, swap chairs with your team members once a week. Even if the chairs are the same make and model, it is a very healthy thing to try someone else's chair.

Change your shoes. When the seasons change, we change our shoes naturally to boots, then back to shoes, then flip flops or sandals. Every time you change your shoes you change the foundation of your body. Be prepared when you go from shoes to sandals to notice some pain or stiffness in your knees, back and even your head. While it is good to be able to switch out your footwear for style, definitely get rid of your shoes when they are too old to support you.

Add orthotics to your shoes. This is the answer to the problem above. You can use custom foot orthotics to keep each shoe feeling the same and supporting you the same. Custom foot orthotics are made from a foam cast of your feet, for your feet. The orthotic inserts help you transition from one pair of shoes to the next with no resultant pain or stiffness in your body because the foundation remains the same.

Stay positive, believe and keep your faith. You have greatness inside you!

For more information please contact me through our website at www.murphyhealthcentre.com. Let me know about your successes and challenges. If you want to share your own awesome healing tips, please share them!

If you or your group would like me to come and speak and share some more healing tips or simply motivate your group or service club, you can contact me through our page here as well: www.murphyhealthcentre.com and click on 'Seminars/ Media'.

Follow our social media links for updates:
Twitter: www.twitter.com/MurphyChiro
Instagram: www.instagram.com/drsean_chiropractor

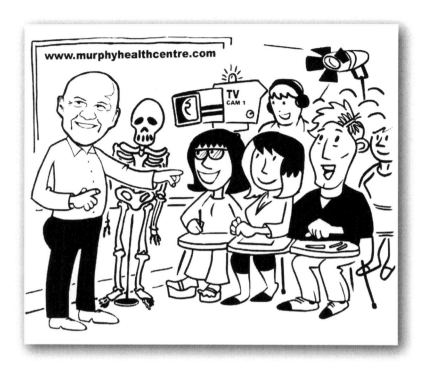

ACKNOWLEDGEMENTS

I would like to lead by example and thank people in Biblical priority order.

First and foremost, I want to thank God for blessing me with the opportunity to serve others. I love people and love caring for their health. You planted the dream in my heart to write a book and this dream is now coming true. Thank you.

Next, I want to thank my awesome wife, Christine for loving me throughout the process of writing this book and everything else we have been through over the past 25 years. I always dream big and could never achieve anything without your undying patience, compassion and love. You are my best friend and companion for life. We do everything together and this book came from your expertise as much as from my own. Let's keep doing life together.

To my awesome children, Rachel and Callum. Thank you for being exactly who you are. God has blessed mom and I with you and we are so proud. You two inspire us daily. You both are the reason I go after my dreams and goals and I love you because you go after yours! You will always be my source of inspiration.

To my mom. You raised me to be strong and focused. Without your amazing upbringing, this book would still be sitting unfinished on the shelf. You are strong, brilliant and funny. You love me, I just know it.

To my sister, Kelly. The humour in this book had me smiling immediately as I wrote it because I could hear your laugh (and some groans) in my head each time I decided to include it. Thank you for being my number one fan and my trusted leader growing up. You taught me style and humour and you taught me to be myself. Thank you.

To my Dad. What can I say? This book is dedicated to you on the first page because you loved this sort of thing. You loved knowing the inside scoop and you would tell EVERYONE about this book if you were still with us. I miss you dearly but you are still with me every day. You are in my curiosity. You are in my love for my family. You are in my fight for what is right. I love you.

In closing, my dad loved blessings and prayers when he was alive. He loved his Irish roots and he loved that my birthday landed on St Patrick's day. In classic Irish prose, I would like to leave you with my Dad's favourite Irish Blessing...

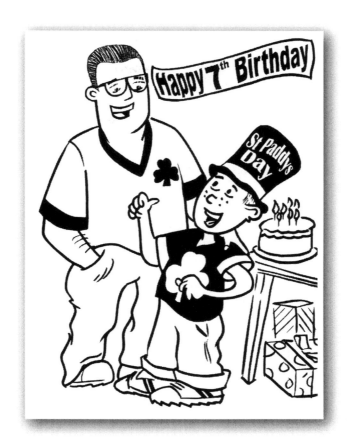

May the road rise up to meet you.
May the wind be always at your back.
May the sun shine warm upon your face.
The rains fall soft upon your fields.
And until we meet again,
May God hold you in the palm of His hand.

Bless you,
Dr. Sean

Notes

Notes

50031337R00057

Made in the USA
Middletown, DE
27 October 2017